HEARING AID PRICES GUIDE 2014

COMPARING PHONAK, WIDEX, SIEMENS, OTICON, STARKEY, RESOUND, UNITRON, DIGITAL HEARING AIDS

Chris Scire

http://www.cshaa.co.uk

Publishers Information

Copyright © 2014 Chris Scire

This edition published in 2014 by Kindle Publishers Pathway

ISBN:1499198701
ISBN-13:978-1499198706

TABLE OF CONTENTS

CHAPTER 1.WHY I WROTE THIS BOOK 4

CHAPTER 2.WHY YOU SHOULD READ THIS BOOK 6

CHAPTER 3.HOW TO BUY A HEARING AID SYSTEM.....................8

CHAPTER 4. HEARING AID PRICES 11

CHAPTER 5. PHONAK HEARING AID PRICES 13

CHAPTER 6. OTICON HEARING AID PRICES 16

CHAPTER 7. WIDEX HEARING AID PRICES 19

CHAPTER 8. STARKEY HEARING AID PRICES 21

CHAPTER 9. GN RESOUND HEARING AID PRICES 23

CHAPTER 10. UNITRON HEARING AID PRICES..........................25

CHAPTER 11. SIEMENS HEARING AID PRICES...........................27

CHAPTER 12. BERNAFON HEARING AID PRICES 29

CHAPTER 13. HEARING AID RETAILERS 31

CHAPTER 14. A FANTASTIC OFFER! 34

CHAPTER 15.ABOUT THE AUTHOR.............................35

CHAPTER 1.

WHY I WROTE THIS BOOK

Many consumers are faced with the problem of where to start when looking to purchase private hearing aids. Where do you go to get a private hearing aid system? Who can you trust for the best prices and service?

It can be a mine field.

Most people when looking for information, would probably search the internet, possibly for many hours, and request information from as many internet sites that they could find.

Some others might ask any friends that they knew who already wore hearing aids and ask them where they got them from and if possible how much they paid for them.

Still others might pop into a couple of High Street retailers and try to find out how much hearing aids were to buy.

It can be a daunting, time consuming process just to find out the best prices to pay for hearing aids.

When they do find out the price of a provider, they spend more than they have to by only sticking with that one provider.

I wrote this book because I wanted to make it easier for people to know exactly how much private digital hearing aids cost and where they can get them from – at the very best prices.

CHAPTER 2.

WHY YOU SHOULD READ THIS BOOK

This book will help you to have an idea as to how much you should pay for private digital hearing aids. The book will also act a guide to help you, the consumer, when seeking to buy a hearing system and what to look out for.

So, you should read this book to save you time. You do not have to spend many hours of searching the internet or walking the High St to find out how much digital hearing aids cost.

You should read this book to save you money – lots of it. You will know what to do in order to avoid the costly mistakes that many have made in purchasing a hearing aid system.

You should read this book because you will avoid the mistakes made by others. Purchasing a new hearing aid system should be a positive life changing experience. Better hearing opens up the world of sound so that you can hear life again. You do not want the purchasing process to be full of regrets.

With this in mind, this brief guide will arm the consumer with the appropriate advice so that they will not have to pay more than is reasonable and will have less chance of being exploited or ripped off.

CHAPTER 3.

HOW TO BUY A HEARING AID

The following points are not meant to be an exhaustive list but more to act as a means of guidance to ensure the main things are covered.

1.Do Shop Around.

It may seem an obvious point but research has shown that nearly 90% of hearing aid purchases take place where the customer has only been to **one** hearing aid specialist.

2.People Buy From People.

Many people purchase a hearing aid system because they like the dispenser. After all they are the one who is going to look after your hearing health. With this in mind, what kind of person are they? Are they professional? Are they a Registered Hearing Aid Audiologist? Are they patient centred or sale centred? Do they have all the necessary equipment to carry out a proper hearing test? What trial period do they offer? Do they explain all the options available and explain all the associated costs involved? Will they provide on-going after care and support?

3.Compare Prices.

Do your research and find like for like products and compare their prices. Find out exactly what is included in the price of the hearing aid system, including warranties, insurance,any extra costs. Are there any charges incurred if you want to cancel the order during any trial period?

Please note that some High Street retailers try to avoid the scrutiny of consumer price comparison by putting their own brand on their hearing aids. Always try to find out the manufacturer and the level of technology.

4.Always Obtain A Written Supply Form

It may again seem obvious but it is really important to get everything in writing. Everything that has been promised, supplier's details, the manufacturer's name, the model and style of the hearing aid, the price, the length of any trial period, any associated costs and details of the warranty.

5.Involve Family And Friends.

When going for a test and finding out about your hearing, take someone else with you. Not only will they be there to support you but they can help you by offering a different opinion about the provider. You do not have to make a decision there and then .

You should never be pressured into making a decision. Nor should you make a decision based on emotions because it can be emotional when hearing loss is corrected and you hear properly for the first time in a while or even years. Try to be logical and assess the real benefits of the hearing aids.

CHAPTER 4.

HEARING AID PRICES

How much are private digital hearing aids?

It can be very confusing to find out just how much private digital hearing aids cost. If you approach a high street retailer, they will probably give you a vague price range from a couple of hundred to several thousand pounds. An independent hearing aid provider can generally offer you a wider choice of manufacturer as well as a cheaper price for a comparable hearing aid system.

I have included a 5 Star Rating System for each manufacturer to give you an idea of the average cost involved when purchasing different technology levels including aftercare.

5* Premium Digital Hearing Aids - High St Price Guide £3,000+ Each, Internet Price Guide £1600 + Each

4* Advanced Digital Hearing Aids - High St Price Guide £2200+ Each, Internet Price Guide

£1300 + Each

3* Performance Digital Hearing Aids - High St Price Guide £1700+ Each, Internet Price Guide £1000 + Each

2* Essential Digital Hearing Aids - High St Price Guide £1200+ Each, Internet Price Guide £700 + Each

1* Basic Digital Hearing Aids - High St Price Guide £600+ Each, Internet Price Guide £300 + Each

CHAPTER 5.

PHONAK HEARING AID PRICES

Phonak are one of the world's largest manufacturers of hearing aids. They are a swiss companty founded in 1947, with their Head Office being in Stafa, Switzerland. In the UK it is based in Warrington where they make all their custom products from. Being a global leader in digital hearing aids means that they are always striving to produce the best hearing aids. Since the release of their first digital hearing aid in 1999, they have progressed to producing the world's smallest bluetooth compatible hearing aid. This is the Phonak Audeo-312.

Phonak hearing aid prices are listed below:

Manufacturer	Hearing Aid	Approx. Internet Prices	Star Rating
Phonak	Bolero / Virto Q90 – inc Nano	£1,595.00	5
Phonak	Bolero / Virto Q70 – inc Nano	£1,295.00	4

Phonak	Bolero / Virto Q50	£995.00	3
Phonak	Virto Nano Q50 Including a 5 Yr Warranty	£1,095.00	3
Phonak	Bolero / Virto Q30	£695.00	2
Phonak	Audeo Q90-10/312/312T	£1,595.00	5
Phonak	Audeo Q70-10/312/312T	£1,295.00	4
Phonak	Audeo Q50-10/312/312T	£995.00	3
Phonak	Audeo Q30-10/312/312T	£645.00	2
Phonak	Naida Q90-UP/SP/CRT	£1,595.00	5
Phonak	Naida Q70-UP/SP/CRT	£1,295.00	4
Phonak	Naida Q50-UP/SP/CRT	£995.00	3
Phonak	Naida Q30-	£645.00	2

	UP/SP/CRT		
Phonak	CROS/BICROS (ITE)	£795 + Cost Of Aid	N/A
Phonak	CROS/BICROS (BTE)	£795 + Cost Of Aid	N/A
Phonak	Accessories Are Available	Various Prices	N/A

CHAPTER 6.

OTICON HEARING AID PRICES

Oticon are a danish company founded in 1904 by Mr Hans Demant. He was determined to produce hearing aids that would be beneficial to their customers. Their worldwide Head Office is in Copenhagen, Denmark. They are currently owned by William Demant Holding. In the UK, all their custom made hearing aids are produced in Hamilton, Scotland.. Oticon uses the latest techniques which includes 3-D modeling and laser moulding technology. Oticon launched their first fully digital hearing aids in 1996. Since then they have established a reputation of being one of the worlds best developers of hearing aid technology.

Oticon hearing aid prices are listed below:

Manufacturer	Hearing Aid	Approx. Internet Prices	Star Rating
Oticon	Alta Pro (H330) – Replaces Agil Pro	£1,595.00	5

Oticon	Alta (H310) – Replaces Agil	£1,495.00	4
Oticon	Nera Pro (H160) – Replaces Acto Pro	£1,095.00	3
Oticon	Nera (H150) – Replaces Acto	£995.00	3
Oticon	Ino Pro (K90)	£695.00	2
Oticon	Ino (K70)	£595.00	1
Oticon	Intega 10 (D100) RIC And Invisible-In-The-Canal	£1,495.00	4
Oticon	Intega 8 (D80) RIC And Invisible-In-The-Canal	£1,295.00	3
Oticon	Intega 6 (D60) RIC Only	£1,095.00	3
Oticon	Chilli SP9 (HH PW70)	£1,495.00	5
Oticon	Chilli SP7 (HH PW50)	£1,195.00	4

Oticon	Chilli SP5 (HH PW30)	£895.00	3
Oticon	Accessories Are Available	Various Prices	N/A

CHAPTER 7.

WIDEX HEARING AID PRICES

Widex was founded by former Oticon employees Eric Westermann and Christian Topholm in 1956. it has remained a family owned business with its Head Office in Allerod, north of Copenhagen. Their UK base is now at Warrington. Widex were the first to release the world's first fully digital hearing aid and have been a world leader since. They currently have the world's smallest receiver-in-canal hearing aid called the Widex Passion.

Widex hearing aid prices are listed below:

Manufacturer	Hearing Aid	Approx. Internet Prices	Star Rating
Widex	Dream 440 – Passion / Fusion / ITE	£1,695.00	5
Widex	Dream 330 – Passion / Fusion / ITE	£1,395.00	4
Widex	Dream 220 – Passion / Fusion /	£1,195.00	3

	ITE		

Widex	Dream 110 – Passion / Fusion / ITE	£995.00	2
Widex	Menu 10 IIC – Invisible Hearing Aids	£1,495.00	5
Widex	Menu 5 IIC – Invisible Hearing Aids	£1,195.00	3
Widex	Menu 3+ IIC – Invisible Hearing Aids	£795.00	2
Widex	Super 440	£1,695.00 +Shell	5

CHAPTER 8.

STARKEY HEARING AID PRICES

Starkey are an American owned company which was first established in 1967 by Mr William Austin. He started it as a hearing aid repair company but it has since grown to be the world's largest manufacturer of custom hearing aids. In the USA and one of the market leaders in Europe. Head office is in Minnesota, USA with its UK offices being based at Stockport. Starkey started to supply digital hearing aids from 1999 and is currently striving to compete with the other manufacturers for market share in Europe.

Starkey hearing aid prices are listed below:

Manufacturer	Hearing Aid	Approx. Internet Prices	Star Rating
Starkey	Soundlens IQ110 IIC- Invisible Hearing Aids	£1,795.00	5
Starkey	Soundlens IQ70 IIC- Invisible	£1,245.00	4

	Hearing Aids		

Starkey	Wi Series 110 / 3 Series 110 / Xino 110	£1,595.00	5
Starkey	Wi Series 90 / 3 Series 90 / Xino 90	£1,295.00	4
Starkey	Wi Series 70 / 3 Series 70 / Xino 70	£1,095.00	3
Starkey	3 Series 30 / Xino 30	£795.00	2
Starkey	3 Series 20 / Xino 20	£595.00	1
Starkey	Accesories Are Available	Various Prices	3

CHAPTER 9.

GN RESOUND HEARING AID PRICES

The name originated from a combination of "Great Nordic" (GN), which was founded in 1895 and "Resound" which was founded as Danovox in 1943 by Mr Gert Rosenstand. The GN Resound group now has over 4600 employees worldwide and its Head Offices are based in Copenhagen, Denmark.

In 2003, GN Resound launched the first fully open-fit hearing aid with the Resound Air (also known as the Contact Air). Resound have since then been active launching a number of innovative products, the latest of which is the world's first iPhone compatible hearing aid called the Resound LiNX

GN Resound hearing aid prices are listed below:

Manufacturer	Hearing Aid	Approx. Internet Prices	Star Rating
GN Resound	LiNK 9 - "Made For iPhone"	£1,650.00	5
GN Resound	LiNK 7- "Made For iPhone"	£1,295.00	4

GN Resound	Verso 9	£1,595.00	5
GN Resound	Verso 7	£1,295.00	4
GN Resound	Verso 5	£995.00	3
GN Resound	Alera 9 – Wireless + £100	£1,395.00	5
GN Resound	Alera 7– Wireless + £100	£1,095.00	4
GN Resound	Alera 5– Wireless + £100	£795.00	3
GN Resound	Alera 4	£745.00	2
GN Resound	Lex 8	£1,395.00	4
GN Resound	Lex 4	£1,095.00	3
GN Resound	Vea 3	£795.00	3
GN Resound	Vea 2	£695.00	2
GN Resound	Vea 1	£595.00	1
GN Resound	Sparx – Power BTE	£895.00	2

GN Resound	Accessories Are Available	Various Prices	N/A

CHAPTER 10.

UNITRON HEARING AID PRICES

Unitron are a canadian company that started about 40 years ago but are now owned by Sonova Holding AG with their head Offices being located in Kitchener, Ontario. Their UK Offices are based in Warrington together with Phonak and all their custom in the ear products are made there. With the backing of the Sonova Group, both companies have been allowed to grow and develop different strategies with regards to hearing aid development. Unitron is not a bit part player in the industry as it employs 600 people worldwide and distributes into over 70 countries.

Unitron hearing aid prices are listed below:

Manufacturer	Hearing Aid	Approx. Internet Prices	Star Rating
Unitron	Quantum2 Pro / Moxi Pro	£1,595.00	5
Unitron	Quantum2 / Moxi 20 / Max 20 Power	£1,495.00	4

Unitron	Quantum2 12 / Moxi 12	£1,195.00	3
Unitron	Quantum2 6/ Moxi 6 / Max 6 Power	£895.00	2
Unitron	Quantum2 E / Moxi E / Max E Power	£595.00	1
Unitron	Tandem 16 CROS / BICROS	£1,495.00	4
Unitron	Tandem 4 CROS / BICROS	£1,195.00	2
Unitron	Accessories are Available	Various Prices	N/A

CHAPTER 11.

SIEMENS HEARING AID PRICES

The German based company is probably the largest supplier of hearing aids in the world. With the Siemens Group behind them, they have the resources to be the most innovative of all the leading hearing aid manufacturers. This is borne out by their pioneering hearing aid technology being used by other manufacturers. This pioneering spirit was evidenced early on in the company's development when Mr Werner von Siemens developed the Phonophor hearing instrument more than a century ago. Siemens released their first fully digital hearing aid in 1996. Since then, they have developed some very innovative products including the Micon chip which has a processing speed of 250 million processes per second.

Siemens hearing aid prices are listed below:

Manufacturer	Hearing Aid	Approx. Internet Prices	Star Rating
Siemens	Micon 7-Pure / Ace / Life / Insio / Motion / Aquaris / Nitro	£1,595.00	5

Siemens	Micon 5-Pure / Ace / Life / Insio / Motion / Aquaris	£1,395.00	4
Siemens	Micon 3- Pure / Life / Motion / Aquaris / Nitro	£1,145.00	3
Siemens	Orion – RIC / S / M / P / ITE	£895.00	2
Siemens	Sirion - RIC / S / M / P / ITE	£645.00	1
Siemens	Imini - 701 – IIC Invisible Hearing Aids	£1,595.00	5
Siemens	Imini – 301 – IIC Invisible Hearing Aids	£1,195.00	3
Siemens	Accessories Are Available	Various Prices	N/A

CHAPTER 12.

BERNAFON HEARING AID PRICES

Bernafon are a swiss company founded in 1946, who are owned by William Demant Holding. Their head Office is located in Bern, Switzerland along with their development and research centre. In the UK, they make all their custom made hearing aids at their UK base located at Hamilton, Scotland. Inspite of having a smaller representation in the UK than Oticon, they still manage to have an impressive innovative product portfolio. They have been able to develop single channel technology that has fast acting compression working alongside multi-channel features.

Bernafon hearing aid prices are listed below:

Manufacturer	Hearing Aid	Approx. Internet Prices	Star Rating
Bernafon	Acriva 9 / Chronos 9	£1,595.00	5
Bernafon	Acriva 7 / Chronos 7	£1,395.00	4
Bernafon	Carista 5 / Chronos 5	£1,195.00	3
Bernafon	Carista 3 / Inizia 3	£895.00	2

Bernafon	Inizia 1	£595.00	1
Bernafon	Accessories Are Available	Various prices	N/A

CHAPTER 13.

HEARING AID RETAILERS

It is generally not known that most of the hearing aid retailers in the UK are owned or affiliated to certain manufacturers.

These relationships need to be borne in mind when visiting the retailer because any recommendation or hearing solution offered is going to be biased toward a certain manufacturer. There is nothing wrong with the hearing aids being recommended. It is just that you might not be given a recommendation from as wide a choice as possible.

You will tend to find Boots Hearing Care (actually David Ormerod Hearing Centres) will recommend Phonak hearing aids.

Hidden Hearing will tend to recommend Oticon hearing aids.

Regional Hearing Services (or Bloom Hearing) will tend to offer Widex hearing aids.

The Hearing Company will tend to dispense Siemens hearing aids.

Amplifon will generally recommend GNResound hearing aids.

Watch out for any special offers because the High St retailer has high prices to start with when compared with a local independent dispenser. So check that the special offer really does offer value for money.

Just a note about Specsavers Hearcare. They provide their own branded hearing aids, making it difficult to know what make is being recommended. This also means that older technology can be offered at a discounted price. Please bear in mind that they also put a "lock" on the hearing aids which means that no one else can alter the programs or settings.

By far the best way to purchase a hearing aid system is to do so through a local independent retailer. By nature these are small to medium sized businesses with lower overheads meaning that these savings can be passed on to the consumer. Being independent also means they are not tied to one particular manufacturer and so tend to give the widest choice of hearing aid solutions on offer. It is vital to check that all hearing aid audiologists are fully qualified and registered with the Health and Care Professions Council (HCPC).

Many independents are members of professional bodies as well. One of the most supported being BSHAA – British Society of Hearing Aid Audiologists.

As an independent myself, I am regularly dispensing hearing aids at 50% off or more than the High Street retailers. I can supply hearing aids at the low internet prices stated in this guide and from all the main manufacturers. My desire is to save you time and money. The feedback I receive from my patients shows that they like my professional patient centred approach and the savings they make as well.

I run my clinics on Tuesdays, Thursdays and Saturdays from the Discount Hearing Aid Centre Row G Leeds City Market (Kirkgate Market) Leeds West Yorkshire LS2 7HY. Tel : 0113 271 4974.

CHAPTER 14.

A FANTASTIC OFFER!

I hope that you have found this guide useful and as a thank you for reading it, I want to make you a very special , limited offer.

Save £100's Even £1000's

A Fantastic 67% Off

High Street Prices

Applies To

5* & 4* Rated Hearing Aids

With This Coupon*

*Terms and Conditions apply

1.Only one voucher per person.

2.You must use and quote the Coupon Code HAP1.

3.The hearing test fee is a non-refundable £25.

4.This offer is subject to change at any time.

CHAPTER 15.

ABOUT THE AUTHOR

My name is Chris Scire, and for the past 10 years I have been a professionally qualified registered hearing aid audiologist.This includes being a Fellow of the British Society of Hearing Aid Audiologists and registered with the Health Care Professions Council.Over those years I have built up a good reputation within the industry. I was very successful as a branch manager with a national company before setting up my own practice. I was a finalist in the "Audiologist Of The Year 2012" competition out of over 500 UK audiologists.

I have met many people from all walks of life over the years and have experience in dealing with people's problems and frustrations. My philosophy is patient centred dispensing. This is carried out in a friendly personal consultative style, where nothing is too much trouble. I have very competitively priced hearing aid solutions for you. I back this up with my no quibble 60 day money back guarantee and free aftercare for the life of the hearing aids. I don't use sales tactics to sell you the most expensive hearing aids.

If you have a question or just want a friendly chat, just contact me at chris@cshaa.co.uk

I look forward to hearing from you.

Kind regards

Chris

Rev Chris Sciré BA PGCE DIPTH RHAD FSHAA

One Last Thing...

If you enjoyed this book or found it useful, I would appreciate it if you would post a short review on Amazon. Your support really does make a difference and I read all the reviews personally so I can get your feedback and make this book even better.

If you would like to leave a review then all you need to do is visit the review link on Amazon here:

In the UK   http://www.amazon.co.uk/HEARING-AID-PRICES-GUIDE-2014-ebook/dp/B00JAJGFSI

In the US   http://www.amazon.com/HEARING-AID-PRICES-GUIDE-2014-ebook/dp/B00JAJGFSI

Thanks again for your support!

The End

.